8 WEEK FITNESS AND NUTRITION JOURNAL

Created by Erika Mitchener
and
Designed by Lois Eastlund

- Follow @plantpowerbootcamp for tips and motivation
- Post your progress using #plantpowerbootcamp
- Visit www.plantpowerbootcamp.com for more details

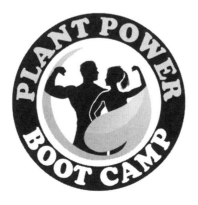

www.plantpowerbootcamp.com
#plantpowerbootcamp ©2019

START

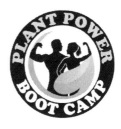

Date: / /

BODY COMPOSITION

WEIGHT: **HIPS:**   **WAIST:**   **CHEST:**   **THIGH:**

PUSH-UP TEST: *How many push-ups can I do in 1 minute?*

PLANK TEST: *How long can I hold plank?*

GOALS

www.plantpowerbootcamp.com
#plantpowerbootcamp ©2019

VEGAN FOOD LOG

Date: / /   Week 1 Day 1

BREAKFAST

LUNCH

DINNER

SNACKS:

WATER:

OTHER:

www.plantpowerbootcamp.com
#plantpowerbootcamp ©2019

FITNESS LOG

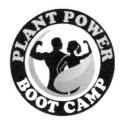

STRENGTH

EXERCISE	SETS	REPS	WT	REST	NOTES

CARDIO

TYPE:

DURATION:

INTENSITY:

OTHER

YOGA/PILATES/STRETCHING/ETC.

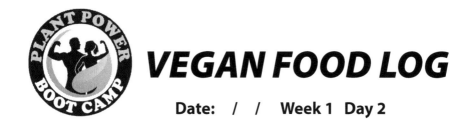

VEGAN FOOD LOG

Date: / / Week 1 Day 2

BREAKFAST

LUNCH

DINNER

SNACKS:

WATER:

OTHER:

FITNESS LOG

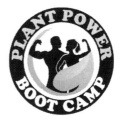

STRENGTH

EXERCISE	SETS	REPS	WT	REST	NOTES

CARDIO

TYPE:

DURATION:

INTENSITY:

OTHER

YOGA/PILATES/STRETCHING/ETC.

www.plantpowerbootcamp.com
#plantpowerbootcamp ©2019

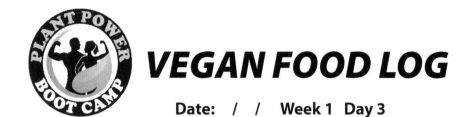

VEGAN FOOD LOG

Date: / / Week 1 Day 3

BREAKFAST

LUNCH

DINNER

SNACKS:

WATER:

OTHER:

FITNESS LOG

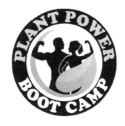

STRENGTH

EXERCISE	SETS	REPS	WT	REST	NOTES

CARDIO

TYPE:

DURATION:

INTENSITY:

OTHER

YOGA/PILATES/STRETCHING/ETC.

www.plantpowerbootcamp.com
#plantpowerbootcamp ©2019

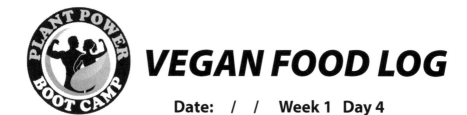

VEGAN FOOD LOG

Date: / /   Week 1 Day 4

BREAKFAST

LUNCH

DINNER

SNACKS:

WATER:

OTHER:

FITNESS LOG

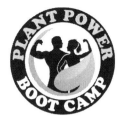

STRENGTH

EXERCISE	SETS	REPS	WT	REST	NOTES

CARDIO

TYPE:

DURATION:

INTENSITY:

OTHER

YOGA/PILATES/STRETCHING/ETC.

www.plantpowerbootcamp.com
#plantpowerbootcamp ©2019

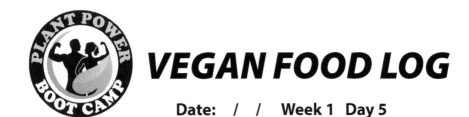

VEGAN FOOD LOG

Date: / /   Week 1 Day 5

BREAKFAST

LUNCH

DINNER

SNACKS:

WATER:

OTHER:

www.plantpowerbootcamp.com
#plantpowerbootcamp ©2019

FITNESS LOG

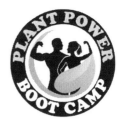

STRENGTH

EXERCISE	SETS	REPS	WT	REST	NOTES

CARDIO

TYPE:

DURATION:

INTENSITY:

OTHER

YOGA/PILATES/STRETCHING/ETC.

www.plantpowerbootcamp.com
#plantpowerbootcamp ©2019

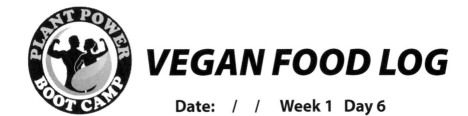

VEGAN FOOD LOG

Date: / / Week 1 Day 6

BREAKFAST

LUNCH

DINNER

SNACKS:

WATER:

OTHER:

FITNESS LOG

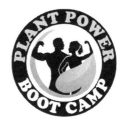

STRENGTH

EXERCISE	SETS	REPS	WT	REST	NOTES

CARDIO

TYPE:

DURATION:

INTENSITY:

OTHER

YOGA/PILATES/STRETCHING/ETC.

www.plantpowerbootcamp.com
#plantpowerbootcamp ©2019

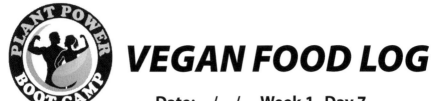

VEGAN FOOD LOG

Date: / / Week 1 Day 7

BREAKFAST

LUNCH

DINNER

SNACKS:

WATER:

OTHER:

FITNESS LOG

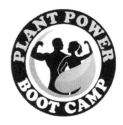

STRENGTH

EXERCISE	SETS	REPS	WT	REST	NOTES

CARDIO

TYPE:

DURATION:

INTENSITY:

OTHER

YOGA/PILATES/STRETCHING/ETC.

www.plantpowerbootcamp.com
#plantpowerbootcamp ©2019

FACTS

"Animal agriculture is responsible for 18 percent of greenhouse gas emissions, more than the combined exhaust from all transportation."

cowspiracy.com/facts

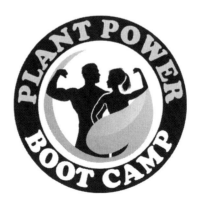

www.plantpowerbootcamp.com
#plantpowerbootcamp ©2019

WEEKLY CHECK IN

WEEK 1

BODY COMPOSITION

WEIGHT: **HIPS:**   **WAIST:**   **CHEST:**   **THIGH:**

PLANK TEST: *How long can I hold plank?*

PUSH-UP TEST: *How many push-ups can I do in 1 minute?*

MINDSET

Did I reach my goals for this week?

What are my goals for the next week?

THOUGHTS:

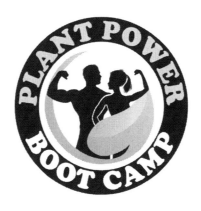

www.plantpowerbootcamp.com
#plantpowerbootcamp ©2019

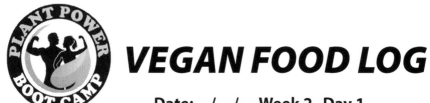

Date: / /   Week 2 Day 1

BREAKFAST

LUNCH

DINNER

SNACKS:

WATER:

OTHER:

www.plantpowerbootcamp.com
#plantpowerbootcamp ©2019

FITNESS LOG

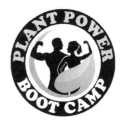

STRENGTH

EXERCISE	SETS	REPS	WT	REST	NOTES

CARDIO

TYPE:

DURATION:

INTENSITY:

OTHER

YOGA/PILATES/STRETCHING/ETC.

www.plantpowerbootcamp.com
#plantpowerbootcamp ©2019

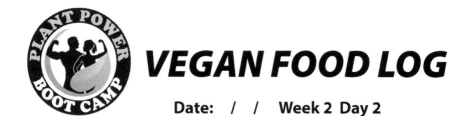

VEGAN FOOD LOG

Date: /   /   Week 2 Day 2

BREAKFAST

LUNCH

DINNER

SNACKS:

WATER:

OTHER:

www.plantpowerbootcamp.com
#plantpowerbootcamp ©2019

FITNESS LOG

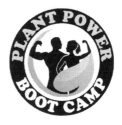

STRENGTH

EXERCISE	SETS	REPS	WT	REST	NOTES

CARDIO

TYPE:

DURATION:

INTENSITY:

OTHER

YOGA/PILATES/STRETCHING/ETC.

www.plantpowerbootcamp.com
#plantpowerbootcamp ©2019

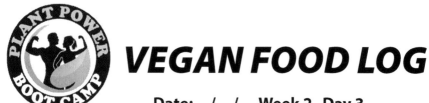

VEGAN FOOD LOG

Date: / /   Week 2 Day 3

BREAKFAST

LUNCH

DINNER

SNACKS:

WATER:

OTHER:

FITNESS LOG

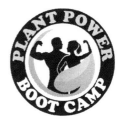

STRENGTH

EXERCISE	SETS	REPS	WT	REST	NOTES

CARDIO

TYPE:

DURATION:

INTENSITY:

OTHER

YOGA/PILATES/STRETCHING/ETC.

www.plantpowerbootcamp.com
#plantpowerbootcamp ©2019

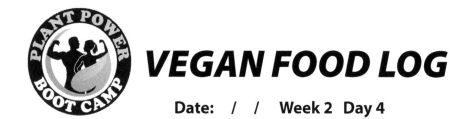

Date: / / Week 2 Day 4

BREAKFAST

LUNCH

DINNER

SNACKS:

WATER:

OTHER:

www.plantpowerbootcamp.com
#plantpowerbootcamp ©2019

FITNESS LOG

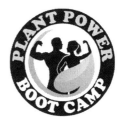

STRENGTH

EXERCISE	SETS	REPS	WT	REST	NOTES

CARDIO

TYPE:

DURATION:

INTENSITY:

OTHER

YOGA/PILATES/STRETCHING/ETC.

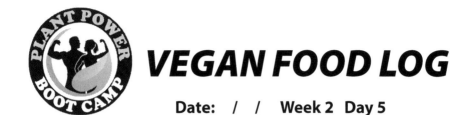

VEGAN FOOD LOG

Date: / / Week 2 Day 5

BREAKFAST

LUNCH

DINNER

SNACKS:

WATER:

OTHER:

www.plantpowerbootcamp.com
#plantpowerbootcamp ©2019

FITNESS LOG

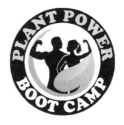

STRENGTH

EXERCISE	SETS	REPS	WT	REST	NOTES

CARDIO

TYPE:

DURATION:

INTENSITY:

OTHER

YOGA/PILATES/STRETCHING/ETC.

www.plantpowerbootcamp.com
#plantpowerbootcamp ©2019

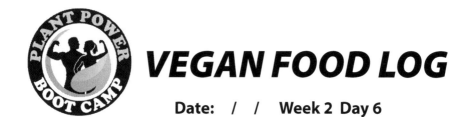

VEGAN FOOD LOG

Date: / /   Week 2 Day 6

BREAKFAST

LUNCH

DINNER

SNACKS:

WATER:

OTHER:

www.plantpowerbootcamp.com
#plantpowerbootcamp ©2019

FITNESS LOG

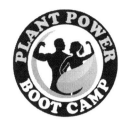

STRENGTH

EXERCISE	SETS	REPS	WT	REST	NOTES

CARDIO

TYPE:

DURATION:

INTENSITY:

OTHER

YOGA/PILATES/STRETCHING/ETC.

www.plantpowerbootcamp.com
#plantpowerbootcamp ©2019

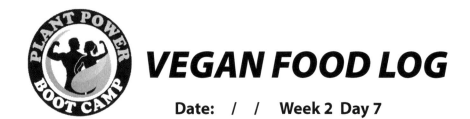

VEGAN FOOD LOG

Date: / /   Week 2 Day 7

BREAKFAST

LUNCH

DINNER

SNACKS:

WATER:

OTHER:

FITNESS LOG

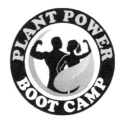

STRENGTH

EXERCISE	SETS	REPS	WT	REST	NOTES

CARDIO

TYPE:

DURATION:

INTENSITY:

OTHER

YOGA/PILATES/STRETCHING/ETC.

www.plantpowerbootcamp.com
#plantpowerbootcamp ©2019

FACTS

"Animal agriculture is responsible for 80-90% of US water consumption."

cowspiracy.com/facts

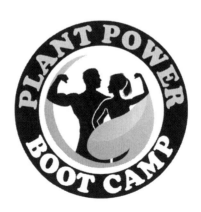

WEEKLY CHECK IN
WEEK 2

BODY COMPOSITION

WEIGHT: **HIPS:**   **WAIST:**   **CHEST:**   **THIGH:**

PLANK TEST: *How long can I hold plank?*

PUSH-UP TEST: *How many push-ups can I do in 1 minute?*

MINDSET

Did I reach my goals for this week?

What are my goals for the next week?

THOUGHTS:

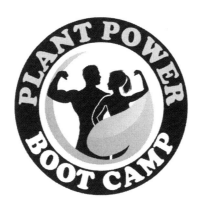

www.plantpowerbootcamp.com
#plantpowerbootcamp ©2019

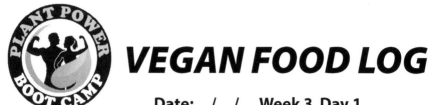

VEGAN FOOD LOG

Date: / /   Week 3 Day 1

BREAKFAST

LUNCH

DINNER

SNACKS:

WATER:

OTHER:

www.plantpowerbootcamp.com
#plantpowerbootcamp ©2019

FITNESS LOG

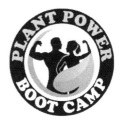

STRENGTH

EXERCISE	SETS	REPS	WT	REST	NOTES

CARDIO

TYPE:

DURATION:

INTENSITY:

OTHER

YOGA/PILATES/STRETCHING/ETC.

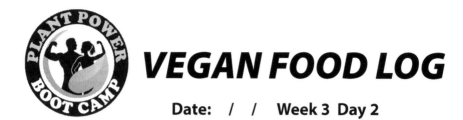

VEGAN FOOD LOG

Date: / /   Week 3 Day 2

BREAKFAST

LUNCH

DINNER

SNACKS:

WATER:

OTHER:

www.plantpowerbootcamp.com
#plantpowerbootcamp ©2019

FITNESS LOG

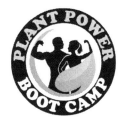

STRENGTH

EXERCISE	SETS	REPS	WT	REST	NOTES

CARDIO

TYPE:

DURATION:

INTENSITY:

OTHER

YOGA/PILATES/STRETCHING/ETC.

www.plantpowerbootcamp.com
#plantpowerbootcamp ©2019

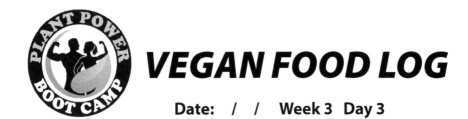

VEGAN FOOD LOG

Date: / /   Week 3 Day 3

BREAKFAST

LUNCH

DINNER

SNACKS:

WATER:

OTHER:

www.plantpowerbootcamp.com
#plantpowerbootcamp ©2019

FITNESS LOG

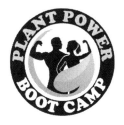

STRENGTH

EXERCISE	SETS	REPS	WT	REST	NOTES

CARDIO

TYPE:

DURATION:

INTENSITY:

OTHER

YOGA/PILATES/STRETCHING/ETC.

www.plantpowerbootcamp.com
#plantpowerbootcamp ©2019

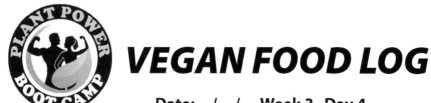

VEGAN FOOD LOG

Date: /   /   Week 3 Day 4

BREAKFAST

LUNCH

DINNER

SNACKS:

WATER:

OTHER:

FITNESS LOG

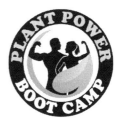

STRENGTH

EXERCISE	SETS	REPS	WT	REST	NOTES

CARDIO

TYPE:

DURATION:

INTENSITY:

OTHER

YOGA/PILATES/STRETCHING/ETC.

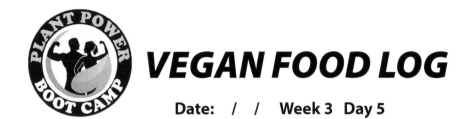

VEGAN FOOD LOG

Date: / / Week 3 Day 5

BREAKFAST

LUNCH

DINNER

SNACKS:

WATER:

OTHER:

www.plantpowerbootcamp.com
#plantpowerbootcamp ©2019

FITNESS LOG

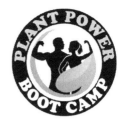

STRENGTH

EXERCISE	SETS	REPS	WT	REST	NOTES

CARDIO

TYPE:

DURATION:

INTENSITY:

OTHER

YOGA/PILATES/STRETCHING/ETC.

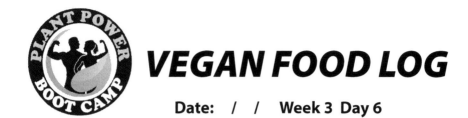

VEGAN FOOD LOG

Date: / /   Week 3 Day 6

BREAKFAST

LUNCH

DINNER

SNACKS:

WATER:

OTHER:

www.plantpowerbootcamp.com
#plantpowerbootcamp ©2019

FITNESS LOG

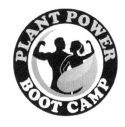

STRENGTH

EXERCISE	SETS	REPS	WT	REST	NOTES

CARDIO

TYPE:
DURATION:
INTENSITY:

OTHER

YOGA/PILATES/STRETCHING/ETC.

www.plantpowerbootcamp.com
#plantpowerbootcamp ©2019

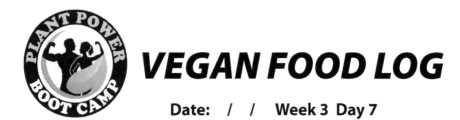

VEGAN FOOD LOG

Date: / /   Week 3 Day 7

BREAKFAST

LUNCH

DINNER

SNACKS:

WATER:

OTHER:

www.plantpowerbootcamp.com
#plantpowerbootcamp ©2019

FITNESS LOG

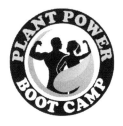

STRENGTH

EXERCISE	SETS	REPS	WT	REST	NOTES

CARDIO

TYPE:

DURATION:

INTENSITY:

OTHER

YOGA/PILATES/STRETCHING/ETC.

FACTS

"2,500 gallons of water are needed to produce 1 pound of beef."

cowspiracy.com/facts

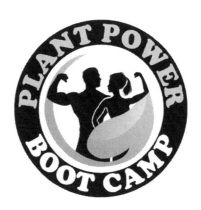

www.plantpowerbootcamp.com
#plantpowerbootcamp ©2019

WEEKLY CHECK IN
WEEK 3

BODY COMPOSITION

WEIGHT: **HIPS:**   **WAIST:**   **CHEST:**   **THIGH:**

PLANK TEST: *How long can I hold plank?*

PUSH-UP TEST: *How many push-ups can I do in 1 minute?*

MINDSET

Did I reach my goals for this week?

What are my goals for the next week?

THOUGHTS:

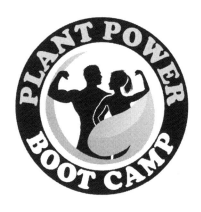

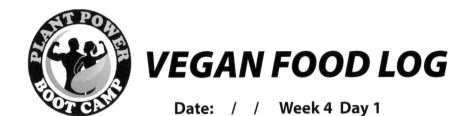

VEGAN FOOD LOG

Date: / /   Week 4 Day 1

BREAKFAST

LUNCH

DINNER

SNACKS:

WATER:

OTHER:

FITNESS LOG

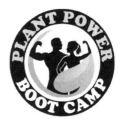

STRENGTH

EXERCISE	SETS	REPS	WT	REST	NOTES

CARDIO

TYPE:

DURATION:

INTENSITY:

OTHER

YOGA/PILATES/STRETCHING/ETC.

www.plantpowerbootcamp.com
#plantpowerbootcamp ©2019

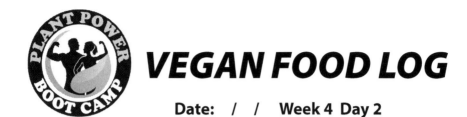

VEGAN FOOD LOG

Date: / / Week 4 Day 2

BREAKFAST

LUNCH

DINNER

SNACKS:

WATER:

OTHER:

FITNESS LOG

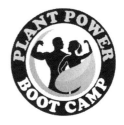

STRENGTH

EXERCISE	SETS	REPS	WT	REST	NOTES

CARDIO

TYPE:

DURATION:

INTENSITY:

OTHER

YOGA/PILATES/STRETCHING/ETC.

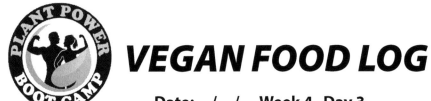

VEGAN FOOD LOG

Date: / /   Week 4 Day 3

BREAKFAST

LUNCH

DINNER

SNACKS:

WATER:

OTHER:

FITNESS LOG

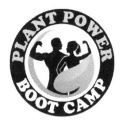

STRENGTH

EXERCISE	SETS	REPS	WT	REST	NOTES

CARDIO

TYPE:

DURATION:

INTENSITY:

OTHER

YOGA/PILATES/STRETCHING/ETC.

www.plantpowerbootcamp.com
#plantpowerbootcamp ©2019

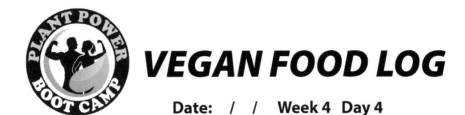

VEGAN FOOD LOG

Date: / / Week 4 Day 4

BREAKFAST

LUNCH

DINNER

SNACKS:

WATER:

OTHER:

FITNESS LOG

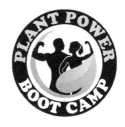

STRENGTH

EXERCISE	SETS	REPS	WT	REST	NOTES

CARDIO

TYPE:
DURATION:
INTENSITY:

OTHER

YOGA/PILATES/STRETCHING/ETC.

www.plantpowerbootcamp.com
#plantpowerbootcamp ©2019

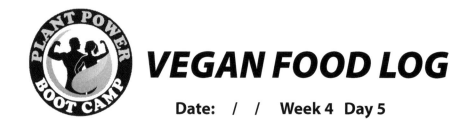

VEGAN FOOD LOG

Date: / /   Week 4 Day 5

BREAKFAST

LUNCH

DINNER

SNACKS:

WATER:

OTHER:

www.plantpowerbootcamp.com
#plantpowerbootcamp ©2019

FITNESS LOG

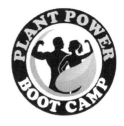

STRENGTH

EXERCISE	SETS	REPS	WT	REST	NOTES

CARDIO

TYPE:

DURATION:

INTENSITY:

OTHER

YOGA/PILATES/STRETCHING/ETC.

www.plantpowerbootcamp.com
#plantpowerbootcamp ©2019

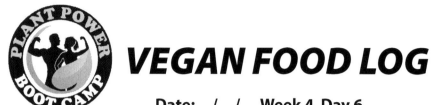

VEGAN FOOD LOG

Date: /   /   Week 4 Day 6

BREAKFAST

LUNCH

DINNER

SNACKS:

WATER:

OTHER:

www.plantpowerbootcamp.com
#plantpowerbootcamp ©2019

FITNESS LOG

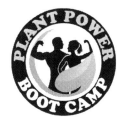

STRENGTH

EXERCISE	SETS	REPS	WT	REST	NOTES

CARDIO

TYPE:
DURATION:
INTENSITY:

OTHER

YOGA/PILATES/STRETCHING/ETC.

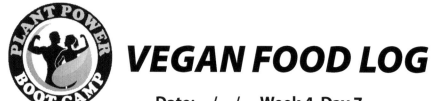

VEGAN FOOD LOG

Date: / / Week 4 Day 7

BREAKFAST

LUNCH

DINNER

SNACKS:

WATER:

OTHER:

www.plantpowerbootcamp.com
#plantpowerbootcamp ©2019

FITNESS LOG

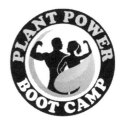

STRENGTH

EXERCISE	SETS	REPS	WT	REST	NOTES

CARDIO

TYPE:

DURATION:

INTENSITY:

OTHER

YOGA/PILATES/STRETCHING/ETC.

www.plantpowerbootcamp.com
#plantpowerbootcamp ©2019

VEGAN CALCULATOR

IN 30 DAYS YOU HAVE SAVED
- *Animal lives: 30*
- *Gallons of water: 33,000*
- *lbs of Co2: 600*

thevegancalculator.com/#calculator

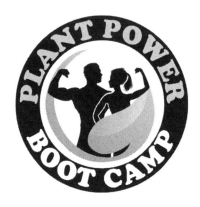

www.plantpowerbootcamp.com
#plantpowerbootcamp ©2019

WEEKLY CHECK IN

WEEK 4

BODY COMPOSITION

WEIGHT: **HIPS:**   **WAIST:**   **CHEST:**   **THIGH:**

PLANK TEST: *How long can I hold plank?*

PUSH-UP TEST: *How many push-ups can I do in 1 minute?*

MINDSET

Did I reach my goals for this week?

What are my goals for the next week?

THOUGHTS:

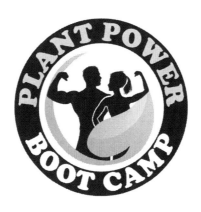

www.plantpowerbootcamp.com
#plantpowerbootcamp ©2019

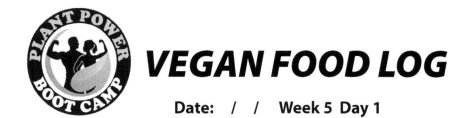

Date: / /   Week 5 Day 1

BREAKFAST

LUNCH

DINNER

SNACKS:

WATER:

OTHER:

FITNESS LOG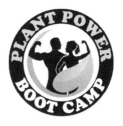

STRENGTH

EXERCISE	SETS	REPS	WT	REST	NOTES

CARDIO

TYPE:

DURATION:

INTENSITY:

OTHER

YOGA/PILATES/STRETCHING/ETC.

www.plantpowerbootcamp.com
#plantpowerbootcamp ©2019

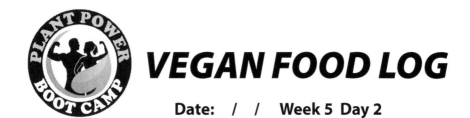

Date: / /   Week 5 Day 2

BREAKFAST

LUNCH

DINNER

SNACKS:

WATER:

OTHER:

FITNESS LOG

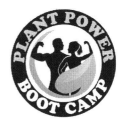

STRENGTH

EXERCISE	SETS	REPS	WT	REST	NOTES

CARDIO

TYPE:

DURATION:

INTENSITY:

OTHER

YOGA/PILATES/STRETCHING/ETC.

www.plantpowerbootcamp.com
#plantpowerbootcamp ©2019

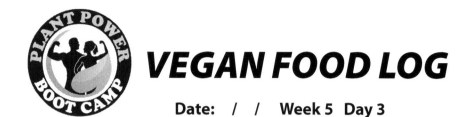

VEGAN FOOD LOG

Date: / / Week 5 Day 3

BREAKFAST

LUNCH

DINNER

SNACKS:

WATER:

OTHER:

FITNESS LOG

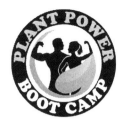

STRENGTH

EXERCISE	SETS	REPS	WT	REST	NOTES

CARDIO

TYPE:

DURATION:

INTENSITY:

OTHER

YOGA/PILATES/STRETCHING/ETC.

www.plantpowerbootcamp.com
#plantpowerbootcamp ©2019

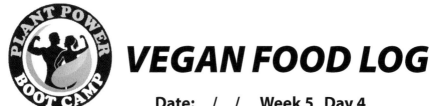

VEGAN FOOD LOG

Date: / / Week 5 Day 4

BREAKFAST

LUNCH

DINNER

SNACKS:

WATER:

OTHER:

www.plantpowerbootcamp.com
#plantpowerbootcamp ©2019

FITNESS LOG

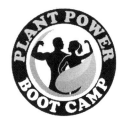

STRENGTH

EXERCISE	SETS	REPS	WT	REST	NOTES

CARDIO

TYPE:

DURATION:

INTENSITY:

OTHER

YOGA/PILATES/STRETCHING/ETC.

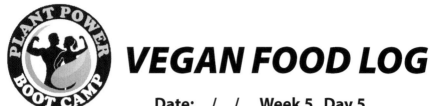

VEGAN FOOD LOG

Date: / /   Week 5 Day 5

BREAKFAST

LUNCH

DINNER

SNACKS:

WATER:

OTHER:

www.plantpowerbootcamp.com
#plantpowerbootcamp ©2019

FITNESS LOG

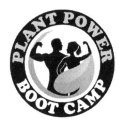

STRENGTH

EXERCISE	SETS	REPS	WT	REST	NOTES

CARDIO

TYPE:

DURATION:

INTENSITY:

OTHER

YOGA/PILATES/STRETCHING/ETC.

www.plantpowerbootcamp.com
#plantpowerbootcamp ©2019

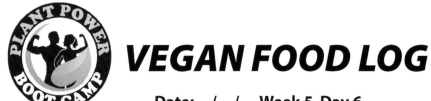

VEGAN FOOD LOG

Date: / /   Week 5 Day 6

BREAKFAST

LUNCH

DINNER

SNACKS:

WATER:

OTHER:

FITNESS LOG

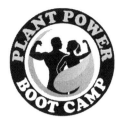

STRENGTH

EXERCISE	SETS	REPS	WT	REST	NOTES

CARDIO

TYPE:

DURATION:

INTENSITY:

OTHER

YOGA/PILATES/STRETCHING/ETC.

www.plantpowerbootcamp.com
#plantpowerbootcamp ©2019

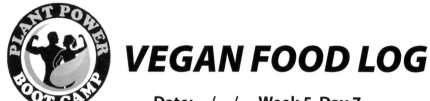

VEGAN FOOD LOG

Date: / /   Week 5 Day 7

BREAKFAST

LUNCH

DINNER

SNACKS:

WATER:

OTHER:

FITNESS LOG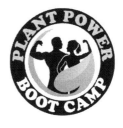

STRENGTH

EXERCISE	SETS	REPS	WT	REST	NOTES

CARDIO

TYPE:

DURATION:

INTENSITY:

OTHER

YOGA/PILATES/STRETCHING/ETC.

FACTS

*"477 gallons of water are required to produce 1lb. of eggs; almost 900 gallons of water are needed for 1lb. of cheese.
1,000 gallons of water are required to produce 1 gallon of milk."*

cowspiracy.com/facts

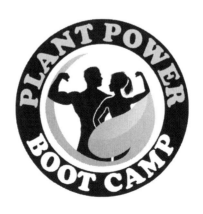

www.plantpowerbootcamp.com
#plantpowerbootcamp ©2019

WEEKLY CHECK IN

WEEK 5

BODY COMPOSITION

WEIGHT:　　**HIPS:**　　**WAIST:**　　**CHEST:**　　**THIGH:**

PLANK TEST: *How long can I hold plank?*

PUSH-UP TEST: *How many push-ups can I do in 1 minute?*

MINDSET

Did I reach my goals for this week?

What are my goals for the next week?

THOUGHTS:

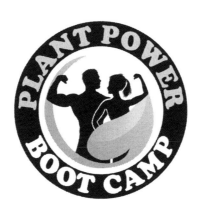

www.plantpowerbootcamp.com
#plantpowerbootcamp ©2019

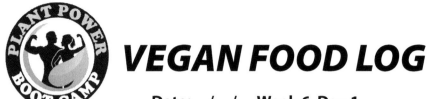

VEGAN FOOD LOG

Date: /   /   Week 6 Day 1

BREAKFAST

LUNCH

DINNER

SNACKS:

WATER:

OTHER:

FITNESS LOG

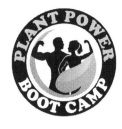

STRENGTH

EXERCISE	SETS	REPS	WT	REST	NOTES

CARDIO

TYPE:

DURATION:

INTENSITY:

OTHER

YOGA/PILATES/STRETCHING/ETC.

www.plantpowerbootcamp.com
#plantpowerbootcamp ©2019

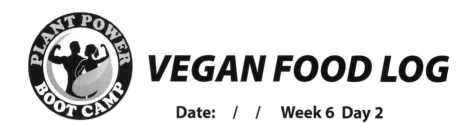

VEGAN FOOD LOG

Date: /   /   Week 6 Day 2

BREAKFAST

LUNCH

DINNER

SNACKS:

WATER:

OTHER:

FITNESS LOG

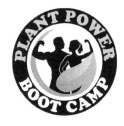

STRENGTH

EXERCISE	SETS	REPS	WT	REST	NOTES

CARDIO

TYPE:

DURATION:

INTENSITY:

OTHER

YOGA/PILATES/STRETCHING/ETC.

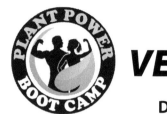

VEGAN FOOD LOG

Date: / /   Week 6 Day 3

BREAKFAST

LUNCH

DINNER

SNACKS:

WATER:

OTHER:

FITNESS LOG

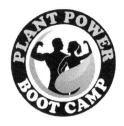

STRENGTH

EXERCISE	SETS	REPS	WT	REST	NOTES

CARDIO

TYPE:
DURATION:
INTENSITY:

OTHER

YOGA/PILATES/STRETCHING/ETC.

www.plantpowerbootcamp.com
#plantpowerbootcamp ©2019

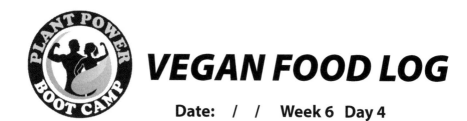

Date: / / Week 6 Day 4

BREAKFAST

LUNCH

DINNER

SNACKS:

WATER:

OTHER:

FITNESS LOG

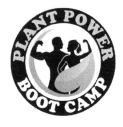

STRENGTH

EXERCISE	SETS	REPS	WT	REST	NOTES

CARDIO

TYPE:
DURATION:
INTENSITY:

OTHER

YOGA/PILATES/STRETCHING/ETC.

www.plantpowerbootcamp.com
#plantpowerbootcamp ©2019

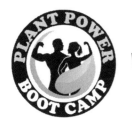

VEGAN FOOD LOG

Date: / /   Week 6 Day 5

BREAKFAST

LUNCH

DINNER

SNACKS:

WATER:

OTHER:

FITNESS LOG

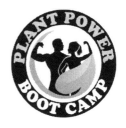

STRENGTH

EXERCISE	SETS	REPS	WT	REST	NOTES

CARDIO

TYPE:

DURATION:

INTENSITY:

OTHER

YOGA/PILATES/STRETCHING/ETC.

www.plantpowerbootcamp.com
#plantpowerbootcamp ©2019

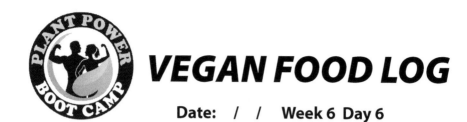

VEGAN FOOD LOG

Date: / / Week 6 Day 6

BREAKFAST

LUNCH

DINNER

SNACKS:

WATER:

OTHER:

FITNESS LOG

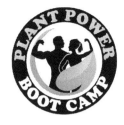

STRENGTH

EXERCISE	SETS	REPS	WT	REST	NOTES

CARDIO

TYPE:

DURATION:

INTENSITY:

OTHER

YOGA/PILATES/STRETCHING/ETC.

www.plantpowerbootcamp.com
#plantpowerbootcamp ©2019

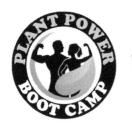

VEGAN FOOD LOG

Date: / /   Week 6 Day 7

BREAKFAST

LUNCH

DINNER

SNACKS:

WATER:

OTHER:

FITNESS LOG

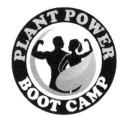

STRENGTH

EXERCISE	SETS	REPS	WT	REST	NOTES

CARDIO

TYPE:
DURATION:
INTENSITY:

OTHER

YOGA/PILATES/STRETCHING/ETC.

www.plantpowerbootcamp.com
#plantpowerbootcamp ©2019

FACTS

*"Land required to feed 1 person for 1 year:
Vegan: 1/6th acre
Vegetarian: 3x as much as a vegan
Meat Eater: 18x as much as a vegan."*

cowspiracy.com/facts

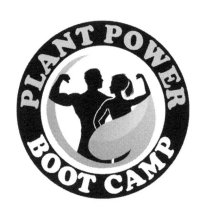

www.plantpowerbootcamp.com
#plantpowerbootcamp ©2019

WEEKLY CHECK IN

WEEK 6

BODY COMPOSITION

WEIGHT: **HIPS:**   **WAIST:**   **CHEST:**   **THIGH:**

PLANK TEST: *How long can I hold plank?*

PUSH-UP TEST: *How many push-ups can I do in 1 minute?*

MINDSET

Did I reach my goals for this week?

What are my goals for the next week?

THOUGHTS:

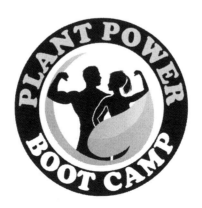

www.plantpowerbootcamp.com
#plantpowerbootcamp ©2019

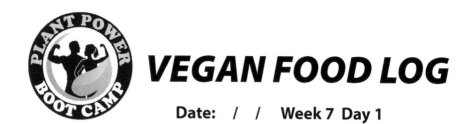

VEGAN FOOD LOG

Date: / /   Week 7 Day 1

BREAKFAST

LUNCH

DINNER

SNACKS:

WATER:

OTHER:

FITNESS LOG

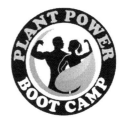

STRENGTH

EXERCISE	SETS	REPS	WT	REST	NOTES

CARDIO

TYPE:

DURATION:

INTENSITY:

OTHER

YOGA/PILATES/STRETCHING/ETC.

www.plantpowerbootcamp.com
#plantpowerbootcamp ©2019

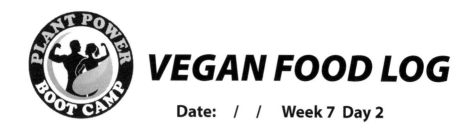

VEGAN FOOD LOG

Date: / /   Week 7 Day 2

BREAKFAST

LUNCH

DINNER

SNACKS:

WATER:

OTHER:

www.plantpowerbootcamp.com
#plantpowerbootcamp ©2019

FITNESS LOG

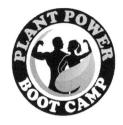

STRENGTH

EXERCISE	SETS	REPS	WT	REST	NOTES

CARDIO

TYPE:

DURATION:

INTENSITY:

OTHER

YOGA/PILATES/STRETCHING/ETC.

www.plantpowerbootcamp.com
#plantpowerbootcamp ©2019

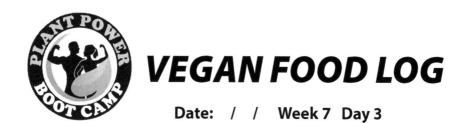

VEGAN FOOD LOG

Date: /   /   Week 7   Day 3

BREAKFAST

LUNCH

DINNER

SNACKS:

WATER:

OTHER:

FITNESS LOG

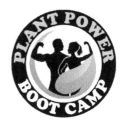

STRENGTH

EXERCISE	SETS	REPS	WT	REST	NOTES

CARDIO

TYPE:

DURATION:

INTENSITY:

OTHER

YOGA/PILATES/STRETCHING/ETC.

www.plantpowerbootcamp.com
#plantpowerbootcamp ©2019

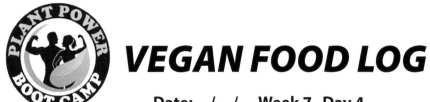

VEGAN FOOD LOG

Date: /   /   Week 7   Day 4

BREAKFAST

LUNCH

DINNER

SNACKS:

WATER:

OTHER:

FITNESS LOG

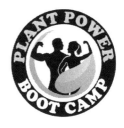

STRENGTH

EXERCISE	SETS	REPS	WT	REST	NOTES

CARDIO

TYPE:

DURATION:

INTENSITY:

OTHER

YOGA/PILATES/STRETCHING/ETC.

www.plantpowerbootcamp.com
#plantpowerbootcamp ©2019

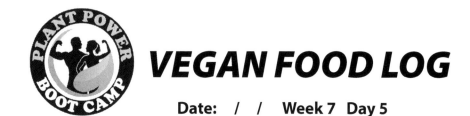

VEGAN FOOD LOG

Date: / /   Week 7 Day 5

BREAKFAST

LUNCH

DINNER

SNACKS:

WATER:

OTHER:

FITNESS LOG

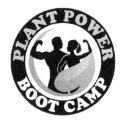

STRENGTH

EXERCISE	SETS	REPS	WT	REST	NOTES

CARDIO

TYPE:

DURATION:

INTENSITY:

OTHER

YOGA/PILATES/STRETCHING/ETC.

www.plantpowerbootcamp.com
#plantpowerbootcamp ©2019

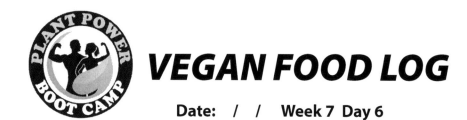

VEGAN FOOD LOG

Date: / / Week 7 Day 6

BREAKFAST

LUNCH

DINNER

SNACKS:

WATER:

OTHER:

FITNESS LOG

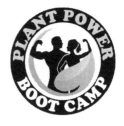

STRENGTH

EXERCISE	SETS	REPS	WT	REST	NOTES

CARDIO

TYPE:

DURATION:

INTENSITY:

OTHER

YOGA/PILATES/STRETCHING/ETC.

www.plantpowerbootcamp.com
#plantpowerbootcamp ©2019

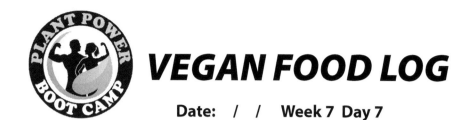

VEGAN FOOD LOG

Date: / / Week 7 Day 7

BREAKFAST

LUNCH

DINNER

SNACKS:

WATER:

OTHER:

FITNESS LOG

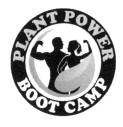

STRENGTH

EXERCISE	SETS	REPS	WT	REST	NOTES

CARDIO

TYPE:

DURATION:

INTENSITY:

OTHER

YOGA/PILATES/STRETCHING/ETC.

FACTS

"82% of starving children live in countries where food is fed to animals, and the animals are eaten by western countries."

cowspiracy.com/facts

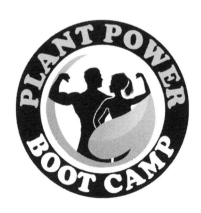

www.plantpowerbootcamp.com
#plantpowerbootcamp ©2019

WEEKLY CHECK IN

WEEK 7

BODY COMPOSITION

WEIGHT: **HIPS:**   **WAIST:**   **CHEST:**   **THIGH:**

PLANK TEST: *How long can I hold plank?*

PUSH-UP TEST: *How many push-ups can I do in 1 minute?*

MINDSET

Did I reach my goals for this week?

What are my goals for the next week?

THOUGHTS:

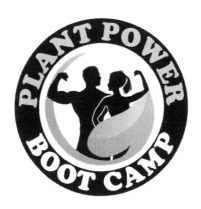

www.plantpowerbootcamp.com
#plantpowerbootcamp ©2019

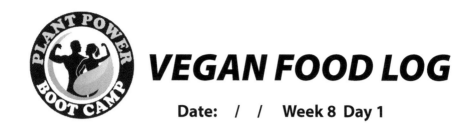

VEGAN FOOD LOG

Date: /   /   Week 8 Day 1

BREAKFAST

LUNCH

DINNER

SNACKS:

WATER:

OTHER:

www.plantpowerbootcamp.com
#plantpowerbootcamp ©2019

FITNESS LOG

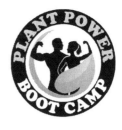

STRENGTH

EXERCISE	SETS	REPS	WT	REST	NOTES

CARDIO

TYPE:

DURATION:

INTENSITY:

OTHER

YOGA/PILATES/STRETCHING/ETC.

www.plantpowerbootcamp.com
#plantpowerbootcamp ©2019

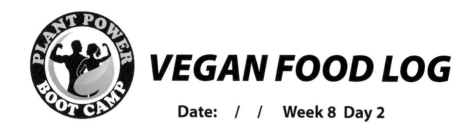

VEGAN FOOD LOG

Date: / /   Week 8 Day 2

BREAKFAST

LUNCH

DINNER

SNACKS:

WATER:

OTHER:

FITNESS LOG

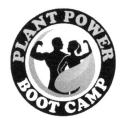

STRENGTH

EXERCISE	SETS	REPS	WT	REST	NOTES

CARDIO

TYPE:

DURATION:

INTENSITY:

OTHER

YOGA/PILATES/STRETCHING/ETC.

www.plantpowerbootcamp.com
#plantpowerbootcamp ©2019

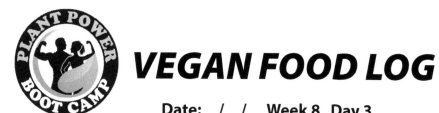

VEGAN FOOD LOG

Date: / / Week 8 Day 3

BREAKFAST

LUNCH

DINNER

SNACKS:

WATER:

OTHER:

FITNESS LOG

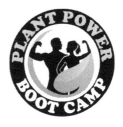

STRENGTH

EXERCISE	SETS	REPS	WT	REST	NOTES

CARDIO

TYPE:

DURATION:

INTENSITY:

OTHER

YOGA/PILATES/STRETCHING/ETC.

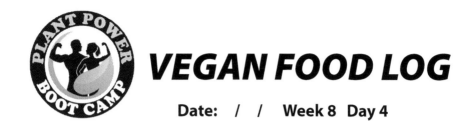

VEGAN FOOD LOG

Date: / /   Week 8 Day 4

BREAKFAST

LUNCH

DINNER

SNACKS:

WATER:

OTHER:

www.plantpowerbootcamp.com
#plantpowerbootcamp ©2019

FITNESS LOG

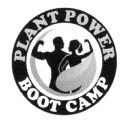

STRENGTH

EXERCISE	SETS	REPS	WT	REST	NOTES

CARDIO

TYPE:

DURATION:

INTENSITY:

OTHER

YOGA/PILATES/STRETCHING/ETC.

www.plantpowerbootcamp.com
#plantpowerbootcamp ©2019

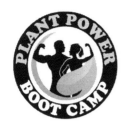

VEGAN FOOD LOG

Date: / /   Week 8 Day 5

BREAKFAST

LUNCH

DINNER

SNACKS:

WATER:

OTHER:

www.plantpowerbootcamp.com
#plantpowerbootcamp ©2019

FITNESS LOG

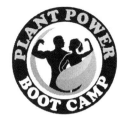

STRENGTH

EXERCISE	SETS	REPS	WT	REST	NOTES

CARDIO

TYPE:

DURATION:

INTENSITY:

OTHER

YOGA/PILATES/STRETCHING/ETC.

www.plantpowerbootcamp.com
#plantpowerbootcamp ©2019

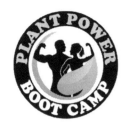

VEGAN FOOD LOG

Date: / / Week 8 Day 6

BREAKFAST

LUNCH

DINNER

SNACKS:

WATER:

OTHER:

www.plantpowerbootcamp.com
#plantpowerbootcamp ©2019

FITNESS LOG

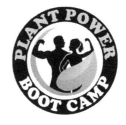

STRENGTH

EXERCISE	SETS	REPS	WT	REST	NOTES

CARDIO

TYPE:

DURATION:

INTENSITY:

OTHER

YOGA/PILATES/STRETCHING/ETC.

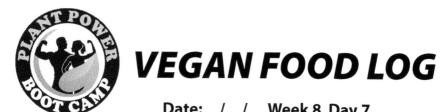

VEGAN FOOD LOG

Date: / /   Week 8 Day 7

BREAKFAST

LUNCH

DINNER

SNACKS:

WATER:

OTHER:

www.plantpowerbootcamp.com
#plantpowerbootcamp ©2019

FITNESS LOG

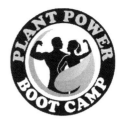

STRENGTH

EXERCISE	SETS	REPS	WT	REST	NOTES

CARDIO

TYPE:

DURATION:

INTENSITY:

OTHER

YOGA/PILATES/STRETCHING/ETC.

www.plantpowerbootcamp.com
#plantpowerbootcamp ©2019

VEGAN CALCULATOR

IN 60 DAYS YOU HAVE SAVED
- Animal lives: 60
- Gallons of water: 66,000
- lbs of Co2: 1200

thevegancalculator.com/#calculator

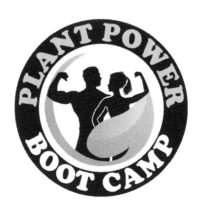

www.plantpowerbootcamp.com
#plantpowerbootcamp ©2019

FINAL CHECK IN

WEEK 8

BODY COMPOSITION

WEIGHT: **HIPS:** **WAIST:** **CHEST:** **THIGH:**

PLANK TEST: *How long can I hold plank?*

PUSH-UP TEST: *How many push-ups can I do in 1 minute?*

MINDSET

Did I reach my goals in these 8 weeks?

What are my future goals?

THOUGHTS:

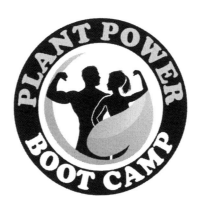

www.plantpowerbootcamp.com
#plantpowerbootcamp ©2019

NOTES

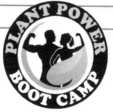

www.plantpowerbootcamp.com
#plantpowerbootcamp ©2019

NOTES

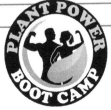

NOTES

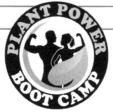

www.plantpowerbootcamp.com
#plantpowerbootcamp ©2019

NOTES

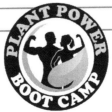

NOTES

Made in the USA
Columbia, SC
12 September 2020